EPSOM
SALT

CARMA
books

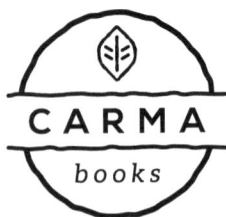

'A conscious approach to health & wellness'

carmabooks.com

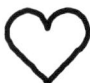

You are invited to to join our **Free Book Club** *mailing list. Sign up via our website to receive* **special offers** *and* **free for a limited time** *Health & Wellness eBooks!*

EPSOM
SALT

♥

50 Miraculous Benefits, Uses & Natural Remedies for Your Health, Body & Home

Carmen Reeves

Disclaimer

This book provides general information and extensive research regarding health and related subjects. The information provided in this book, and in any linked materials is for informational purposes only, and is not intended to be construed as medical advice. Speak with your physician or other healthcare professional before taking any nutritional or herbal supplements. There are no 'typical' results from the information provided - as individuals differ, the results will differ. Before considering any guidance from this book, please ensure you do not have any underlying health conditions which may interfere with the suggested healing methods. If the reader or any other person has a medical concern or pre-existing condition, he or she should consult with an appropriately licensed physician or healthcare professional. Never disregard professional medical advice or delay in seeking it because of something you have read in this book or in any linked materials. The reader assumes the risk and full responsibility for all actions, and the author or publisher will not be held liable for any loss or damage that may result from the information presented in this publication.

Carma Books
carmabooks.com

hello@carmabooks.com

CONTENTS

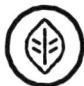

INTRODUCTION

Thank you for your purchase of *'Epsom Salt: 50 Miraculous Benefits, Uses & Natural Remedies for Your Health, Body & Home'*. This book will be your guide to learning more about a seemingly simple, everyday product that can vastly improve your mind, body, health and home.

Not quite convinced? Well consider that the medicinal benefits of Epsom salts have been practiced for hundreds of years, and even today, people all over the world use them for a variety of ailments and everyday tasks. Perhaps you are struggling with a certain health problem, a garden that is lacking, or you just want to know more about this all-natural, traditional substance that your grandma used to add to her bathtub.

You will find it all in this helpful guide. Epsom salts may rescue you from a yo-yo diet, a chronic and debilitating health woe or hours wasted on perfecting your house-hold-cleaning routine. Just read on and see what all the fuss is about; this book may become your new go-to manual for many of the issues – big and small – that life throws at you.

Best of all, you can easily find Epsom salt in your local convenience store, supermarket or drugstore. Plus, it's an affordable option that will save you from those expensive spa treatments or chemical-laden home and beauty products. There is no excuse not to take advantage of this helpful multi-purpose mineral! *Here is what you can expect from this book:*

An introduction to Epsom salt and its history.
First-aid applications: From small boo-boos to bigger issues, Epsom salts can help!

Beauty benefits: Seeking smoother, more radiant skin? Softer, kissable lips? Or perhaps healthier hair? Find all that and more with Epsom salts.

Improve your health: The multiple health advantages of Epsom salts, including remedies that are super easy and simple to use.

Handy for household chores: Even your home can benefit from this wondrous mineral – from cleaning bathroom tiles to softening fabric – Epsom salt has you covered.

Great garden uses: Amp up your gardening regimen with a variety of all natural quick-fixes.

Wonderful for weight loss: Did you know that using Epsom salt can even help shift those extra pounds?

Soothing sea baths: Use Epsom salt in your bath time routine for a variety of healing properties. Just read on to discover the numerous benefits!

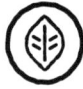

CHAPTER 1

What is Epsom Salt?

Surprisingly, Epsom salt is not even a salt at all! It is however, a naturally occurring mineral, known as magnesium sulfate, that was discovered hundreds of years ago in a water spring in Epsom, a village in Surrey, England (hence its name, Epsom salt).

Epsom salt was prepared by boiling down spring water, which contained porous chalk material from North Downs (UK) combined with non-porous clay silt from London. This treatment and chemical reaction resulted in the crystal-like mineral we now refer to as Epsom salts – a match made in heaven. Now, a process using magnesium and sulfur treated together creates the compound, Epsom salt, we commonly find in stores.

For a while, Epsom salt was solely used by farmers who wanted to improve their crop yield; then by the end of the 1970's, over 2 million tons of the mineral was being used all around the world. After common use, other applications for Epsom salts also became popular, one of them being its use as a drying agent. Since the mineral is quick to take in moisture, bacteria and condensation, Epsom salt was commonly used by doctors and medical professionals to sanitize or prepare medical tools and instruments. Because of its multitude of uses, Epsom salt has received the prestigious honor of being included in the *World Health Organization's Model List of Essential Medicines.*

As for mainstream society and those outside of the medical field, Epsom salt was (and still is) commonly used for bathing – much like a 'traditional' bath salt. Since magnesium sulfate is able to effectively ease aches and pains, it is a favorite amongst athletes and those with chronic body pain and discomfort as an easy and affordable mode of pain relief.

Now people all over the world use this all-natural product for a variety of uses, and it isn't purely for tradition's sake. Even numerous studies have demonstrated Epsom salt's amazing and wide-ranging benefits.

Why Should I Use Epsom Salt?

So, why should you use Epsom salt? Epsom salts have long been utilized as an all-natural treatment for the **body, mind and soul** – including remedies related to health and medicine, beauty and aesthetics, and home and garden.

In terms of health and medicine, it has been shown that Epsom salts are easily absorbed by our skin, which is why many people prefer to use this mineral as an added luxury to their bathing routine.

Here are just a few of the many uses for Epsom salts, which we will revisit throughout this book:

• Epsom salts **ease stress** and **relax** your mind and body by producing serotonin, a 'happy' chemical in the brain that promotes a feeling of calm and peace.

• Daily stress can drain and deplete your body of various nutrients, including much needed magnesium. Epsom salt, being high in **magnesium** content, is an effective way to absorb and replenish this essential nutrient through the skin.

• With its composition of over 352 different enzymes, Epsom salt has become a valuable health companion in helping reduce the appearance and discomfort related to inflammatory **skin conditions**, such as **rosacea** and **eczema**.

• Those suffering from inflammation such as **debilitating headaches, arthritis, gout, muscle soreness, cramps** or **nerve damage** may find Epsom salt baths to be a beneficial treatment in easing pain, as it helps balance electrolytes in the body.

• Even for more serious health concerns, Epsom salts can **improve artery function, lower blood pressure, improve blood circulation** and reduce the risk of **blood clots**.

• Epsom salts help your body **detoxify** by eliminating and flushing harmful bacteria, toxins and heavy metals from your cells.

But it is not all health and medicine for Epsom salts. **Try using these minerals to improve your skin's overall smoothness and appearance.** With its exfoliating and cleansing properties, there are many people who take advantage of Epsom salts' ability to enhance your skin's radiance.

The magnesium sulfate contained in Epsom salt is also extremely useful when used in the home. You will find that just about every room in your house can benefit from a little application of Epsom salt. For instance, bathroom tiles can get a powerful scrubbing, or your ordinary kitchen cleaner can be revived with the addition of some Epsom salts. Even caring for your home's garden and exterior is easier with the help of this handy mineral.
There are many more uses of Epsom salts and we will touch on these applications throughout this book. So, let's get started in learning more about this mineral and how it can be useful in your everyday life.

Before You Get Started

Although Epsom salt is a natural mineral it is important to use it wisely and with caution, particularly when utilizing it for healthcare. Don't go overboard with Epsom salts; they should only be for occasional use. Start out by using Epsom salt baths twice per week and gradually increase as needed.

Ensure the type of Epsom salt you purchase contains *magnesium sulfate* as its main ingredient. Consult the package for directions and dosage and **do not** use or ingest more than is recommended per day.

If you have any medical conditions or are pregnant, first consult your doctor before using or ingesting Epsom salt. Do not use Epsom salt if you have kidney problems or serious digestive conditions. Do not use Epsom salt on children under 6 years of age. People with diabetes or those with fragile skin are advised to use gentle foot soaks to reap the benefits of Epsom salt, instead of full body soaks.

In some people, the magnesium present in Epsom salt might cause stomach upset or other symptoms when ingested, and if taken in very large amounts can be unsafe and cause serious side effects. Check with your doctor if you suspect you are ill.

Take precautions to ensure your pets **do not** consume Epsom salt.

Always use Epsom salt with care and exercise your own judgment when taking any nutritional supplements.

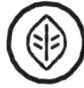

CHAPTER 2

Epsom Salt for Body and Mind

Now that we know more about what Epsom salts are and where they come from, let's take a deeper look at how they can improve your life. Here you will discover how Epsom salts can revamp your beauty routine and come in handy for those everyday fiascos. There really is no reason not to pick up a package of this inexpensive yet valuable mineral.

Sea Bath Recipes

Bathing in a simple mixture of water and Epsom salts is a long-held tradition for many people. You may have heard your grandmother tout the benefits of soaking in an Epsom salt bath. Now you can try it for yourself and discover that she was actually 100% right!

Epsom salt baths have a natural way of easing and relaxing the body, which in turn helps to soothe the mind after a long, busy day. So how does this work? Epsom salt contains magnesium, and it has been shown that when you are stressed out, your body becomes depleted of this essential element. By simply soaking your body in a bath of Epsom salt, you will allow yourself to unwind and effectively replenish the levels of magnesium in your system. Stress also results in increased levels of adrenaline in the body – magnesium boosts serotonin production, which balances out the excess adrenaline in your system.

Did you know that more than half of the adults in the United States have a magnesium deficiency, which could ultimately result in higher stress levels? It's lucky for us that Epsom salts can help us correct this issue.

Besides the mood stabilizing properties of Epsom salt, it can also improve your energy and endurance via the production of adenosine triphosphate (or ATP) in the body. ATP is a huge power-player in your body's cells and plays a big part in how energetic you feel throughout your day. When you pair this with the magnesium ions that are present in Epsom salt, this helps kick up your energy levels a few notches! While the magnesium ions help balance your adrenaline levels, they also decrease other symptoms such as irritability, moodiness and fatigue. In fact, many doctors and experts claim that soaking in a relaxing bath of Epsom salts just a few times per week can result in revitalizing, energizing results. How easy is that?

With a more relaxed mind, you can have more of a restful sleep. Are you tired of tossing and turning at night? Do you wake up feeling as though you've barely slept at all? Try soaking in a soothing Epsom salt bath before bedtime. Your mind will wind down while your muscles and joints feel alleviated. Studies have also shown that your mind can reap just as many benefits from Epsom salt baths as your body, including improved concentration and mental focus.

If you are looking to rid your body of nasty toxins, then a detoxing bath of Epsom salt could do just the trick for you. The main contributing factor in the detoxification process is, once again, the magnesium sulfate in Epsom salt. These crucial elements work overtime to ensure that your bodily systems are operating just as they should. Sulfate is absorbed by your body and helps to build up stronger intestinal walls so that you can more easily release toxins from your system, and paired with magnesium, boosts enzymes found in the pancreas that aid in digestion.

Magnesium sulfate is also useful for clearing out heavy metals from your system, playing a part in the purifying and detoxifying process. To take advantage of these wonderful effects, just fill up your bathtub and mix in one to two cups of Epsom salt. For best results, the water should not be scalding hot but just warm enough for a cozy bath – this will help the Epsom salt to be effectively absorbed by the skin. You can take this bath a few times per week; preferably right before bedtime.

The following is a collection of beautiful bath recipes using the ever-marvelous Epsom salts. **Feel free to alter each recipe depending on what you have on hand** – you may even decide to keep things super simple and use Epsom salt on its own. I have however discovered the value in the following combinations to boost and enhance its incredible healing properties.

♥

1) Skin Soothing Coco-Bath

This relaxing bath will leave you feeling calm, refreshed and moisturized. A combination of Epsom salt and coconut milk is perfect for soothing dry or irritated skin.

Ingredients:
• Epsom salts, 1/2 cup
• Warm water, enough to fill your bathtub
• Can of coconut milk
• Essential oil of your choice, optional *(lavender helps calm irritated skin)*

Directions:
1) Fill bathtub with warm water.

2) Dissolve Epsom salts, add a few drops of essential oil if desired.

3) Add can of coconut milk for a deeper moisturizing effect.

4) Soak in bathtub for 15 minutes.

♥

2) Detoxifying ACV Bath for Headaches

Try this no-hassle detoxifying bath recipe, which draws out toxins and balances your skin's pH levels, and also works wonders for soothing migraines and headaches.

Ingredients:
• Epsom salts, 1/4 cup

• Apple Cider Vinegar, 1/3 cup

• Baking soda, 1/4 cup

• Essential oil of your choice, 5-10 drops *(a blend of both peppermint and lavender aids in headache relief)*

Directions:

1) Dissolve Epsom salts and baking soda in a cup of boiling water.

2) Add apple cider vinegar to a tub-full of warm water.

3) Add the Epsom salt and baking soda mixture to the tub before adding the essential oil.

4) Soak for 30 minutes.

♥

3) Fizzy Bath Bomb for Stress Relief

Want to turn your bath experience into a stress-relieving spa treatment? There's no better way than to create your own bath bombs using these relaxing and detoxifying ingredients – a perfect combination for uplifting your mood and lowering blood pressure.

Ingredients:
• Epsom salts, 1/2 cup

• Baking soda, 1 cup

• Citric acid, 1/2 cup

• Witch hazel, 2 teaspoons

• Olive oil, 2 teaspoons

• Vanilla extract, 1 teaspoon

• Vanilla essential oil, 5-10 drops

Directions:

1) In a bowl, combine baking soda, salts, and citric acid.

2) In a separate container, mix olive oil, witch hazel, vanilla extract, and essential oil.

3) Add the liquid ingredients to the dry ingredients and mix thoroughly using your gloved hand.

4) Pour mixture in your desired greased mold, or greased muffin tin and leave for 24 hours. It will expand and that's normal – you can continue to gently push the mixture into the mold so that it doesn't expand too much.

5) Transfer into air-tight jar or container and use within 2 weeks.

♥

4) Therapeutic Bath Salts

Creating your own bath salt will 'personalize' your relaxation experience, encouraging you to enjoy more of the therapeutic benefits of Epsom salts. Feel free to experiment with your favorite scents and colors for a sensory bath time experience.

Ingredients:

• Epsom salts, 2 cups

• Olive oil, 1 teaspoon

• Essential oil of your choice, 5-10 drops

• All-natural food coloring, 2 drops (optional)

Directions:

1) In a bowl, combine all ingredients and mix well until

evenly distributed.

2) Transfer mixture into an air-tight jar.

3) Add a few tablespoons to your bath and enjoy.

Beauty Benefits

Epsom salts work wonders for your internal body, but what about the outside? Your exterior can be just as healthful as your interior with the help of these Epsom salt beauty recipes. While it is most traditionally used in baths, it can also be used and applied while showering. You may already be familiar with the couple of Epsom salt recipes featured in my *Homemade Organic Skin & Body Care* book. Otherwise, you may not have considered including Epsom salts in your beauty routine, but after you discover the beauty benefits of this miraculous mineral, you will be rushing out the door to buy some! From your head to your toes, there are multiple advantages to using Epsom salts for skin care. Your lips, eyes, feet and more will feel flawless after replacing your expensive, store-bought products with Epsom salts.

Epsom salt does not dry out your skin like sea salt can and instead softens your skin without leaving any residue. The moisturizing and exfoliating properties of Epsom salts are highly regarded and an excellent alternative to throwing away out your hard-earned money on expensive beauty treatments. Forget about hitting the pricey spa or salon for a manicure, pedicure or facial treatment. You can have your very own home spa on the cheap, with amazing results. Just hit your local grocery store for an affordable package of Epsom salts.

Each of the following recipes boast different benefits – so be sure to try them all out to explore how such a simple ingredient can drastically improve your skin, hair and body.

5) Exfoliating Body Scrub

Whip up this delightful exfoliating scrub that will leave your skin feeling fresh and tingly from the removal of dead skin cells. The result? Smoother, more radiant skin.

Ingredients:
• Epsom salts, 2 cups

• Olive oil, 2 Tablespoons

• Juice from 1/2 of medium-sized lemon *(or other fruit juice if you have sensitive skin)*

• Herbs of your choice *(try lavender buds or dried rosemary)*

Directions:
1) Combine all the ingredients.

2) Gently massage all over body. You can use it dry or in-shower. If you choose to scrub dry, rinse it afterwards with warm water.

3) Remaining product can be stored in an air-tight jar; use once or twice per week.

6) Purifying Facial Cleanser

You can use Epsom salts on your face as well. All it takes is a small portion of Epsom salts mixed with coconut oil to reveal firmer and smoother skin. The exfoliation boosts magnesium in the skin while adding more hydration and removing toxins.

Simply combine **1 teaspoon** of Epsom salts and **a handful of coconut oil** into a bowl. Use this mixture as an alternative to commercial cleansers. On top of cleansing, this mixture can also aid in repairing your skin from sun damage.

7) Moisturizing Body Butter

Moisturizing after you shower is important if you want to maintain smooth, rejuvenated skin, so allow Epsom salts take care of that for you! Epsom salt contains softening and soothing properties making this luxurious recipe especially helpful for dry skin.

Ingredients:
• Epsom salts, 1/2 cup

• Boiling water, 2 Tablespoons

• Unrefined coconut oil, 1/2 cup

• Candelilla wax, 1 Tablespoon

• Shea butter, 3 Tablespoons

Directions:

1) Mix water and Epsom salts, allow to cool.

2) Combine candelilla wax, shea butter, and coconut oil in a jar and place the jar in a pan with water. Place pan over medium heat and wait until mixture melts.

3) Blend the oil mixture (you can use a hand blender).

4) Slowly add the Epsom salt mixture.

5) Place in fridge for 15 minutes before blending again to get the consistency of a body butter.

8) Blemish & Blackhead Treatment

We all suffer from acne at some point or another. Now you can use Epsom salts to reduce the appearance of pimples, blemishes and blackheads by ridding your skin of bacteria and toxins. Rather than buy expensive cleansers and spot treatments, just try this combination at home – use it as a part of your regular skin-care routine and you are sure to see results.

Ingredients:
• Epsom salts, 1 Tablespoon

• Hot water, 1 cup

• Iodine, 3 drops

Directions:

1) Boil one cup of water.

2) Combine water, iodine, and Epsom salts.

3) Allow to cool, store in an airtight glass container.

4) Use cotton swab or puff to dab at your blemishes and let it sit for no more than 10 minutes.

5) Rinse well with warm water.

9) Chapped Lip Scrub

Dry, flakey lips are not only annoying, they are also a little unsightly! For softer, more kissable lips, try this super easy recipe. This mixture will give your lips a deep moisturizing treatment while removing dry skin and dead cells.

The recipe is very simple: just combine **1 teaspoon of Epsom salts** and **1 teaspoon of pure maple syrup**. Gently massage the mixture onto your lips in a circular motion and leave for a few minutes before wiping with a damp washcloth. You will notice renewed skin and smoothness instantly!

10) Refreshing Mouth Rinse

It's not just your skin that can be cleansed; you can improve your oral hygiene with Epsom salts as well. Epsom salts act as a natural anti-bacterial, so try this simple remedy to combat bad breath, toothache, or even a sore throat.

Take **2 tablespoons of Epsom salts** and mix it with **a cup of warm water** until dissolved. Gargle mixture for a few minutes, and voila! You have yourself a simple, refreshing mouthwash – *the natural way*.

❤

11) Purifying Pre-Shampoo Rinse

If you like to use styling products in your hair, then you have probably experienced the residue and roughness it leaves behind. Now you can move away from crunchy, dry locks and use Epsom salts to deeply cleanse your hair. This recipe also makes for a fantastic anti-dandruff and oily hair treatment. It's super easy and you can keep this concoction in your bathroom for a simple application whenever you need it.

Ingredients:
• Epsom salts, 1 teaspoon
• Baking soda, 1 teaspoon
• Hot water, 1 cup
• Lemon juice, 1/2 cup

Directions:
1) Combine Epsom salts, lemon juice, baking soda and water. Allow to dissolve and cool.

2) Pour and gently massage mixture into slightly dampened scalp and let it soak for 20 minutes.

3) Rinse thoroughly and follow with regular shampoo routine.

For a variety of all-natural hair care recipes, including shampoos, conditioners and hair masks, you may benefit from my book: *Homemade Natural Hair Care (with Essential Oils)*.

♥

12) Volumizing Conditioner

To create a super simple conditioner that will add more bounce to your tresses, turn to Epsom salts. Aside from adding extra volume to your hair, the salts also act as a natural cleanser and moisturizer, which will add a healthy luster to your locks.

In a small container, combine **2 tablespoons of olive oil** and **3 tablespoons of Epsom salts**; use in replacement of your regular conditioner and notice the results after just a few washes!

♥

13) Soothing Eye Compress

To reduce red, puffy or irritated eyes, try using this simple Epsom salt eye compress. Use this remedy up to three times per week for best results. The magnesium in the salts help soothe pain and fight off any infection – a lifesaver for people with conjunctivitis and cataracts.

Mix **3 tablespoons of Epsom salts** and **3 table-spoons of hot water**. Cool the solution for a few minutes or until temperature is comfortable for you. Soak a clean cloth in the solution and place the cloth over your closed eyes. Leave for 2-3 minutes and rinse well with cold water.

14) Multi-Purpose Foot Soak

Not only are foot soaks a great way to pamper yourself – they are also an effective remedy for pain relief from tired, sore feet, as well as eliminating toe fungus or that pesky foot odor. Professional foot soaks can be expensive and unnecessary when you can easily mix your own Epsom salt foot soak at home. Epsom salts are great for exfoliating skin and will rid your feet of dry, dead skin cells.

Ingredients:

• Epsom salts, 1/2 cup

• Warm water, 1 foot-tub full

• Lemon juice, 1 cup

Optional:

• Essential oils (lavender or tea tree for antibacterial properties)

• Baking soda to soften skin

• Slices of ginger for detoxifying benefits

Directions:

1) Combine Epsom salts, warm water and lemon (and other optional ingredients, if you choose to add any).

2) Dissolve Epsom salts and soak feet for 30-45 minutes. Use this 2-3 times a week, especially at night, after a long day at work.

Forget toting around a clunky first aid kit; all you need are Epsom salts (and water) to relieve some of the most common first-aid fiascos. From bites and stings to splinters and rashes, this little treasure-trove can do it all.

15) Sunburn Soother

We all hate getting sunburn, but if you were less than wise and got burnt, thankfully you can find relief with Epsom salts. This remedy is boasted to be much more effective than aloe treatments and other commercial products. Since magnesium sulfate is an anti-inflammatory compound, it is a wonderful way to ease the effects of red, irritated skin.

In **a cup of water**, stir in **2 tablespoons of Epsom salts**; transfer the mixture into a clean, fine mist spray bottle for easy direct-to-skin application. You can also soak a clean cloth and place it over the affected area.

16) Bee Sting Solution

Bee stings hurt! But luckily you can get quick pain relief with Epsom salts – this solution will minimize swelling and discomfort.

Soak a cotton ball or cotton cloth in **a cup of cold water** with **2 tablespoons of Epsom salts**. Apply directly over the affected skin. Alternatively, if you have been stung in more than one place, you can resort to soaking in an Epsom salt bath **(2 cups of Epsom salts with warm water)** for 12 minutes.

♥

17) Bug Bite Remedy

Bug bites happen all year round, so an on-the-spot remedy should always be in your kit. Skip the inconvenience of visiting your pharmacist and whip up this Epsom salt solution for easy and affordable relief whenever you need it.

Boil **a cup of water** and mix in **a teaspoon of Epsom salts**. To cool it down, place it in the fridge for around 20 minutes. Stir again and then apply the pasty substance directly onto the bug bite. Be sure to clean and dry the affected area first.

♥

18) Splinter Compress

This little-known remedy may save you a trip to the doctor's office to remove that troublesome splinter. Place **a small pinch** of Epsom salt to the affected area and cover with a band-aid. Change the band-aid once per day with the Epsom salt application. After a couple of days, you will hopefully notice the splinter stick out through the skin – carefully use tweezers to pull it out.

You may also use an Epsom salt cooling compress after you finally get that pesky splinter out. The compress will help to soothe the swelling and inflammation that often results after you pull out a splinter. This will prevent your skin from getting more irritated. Mix **a cup of cold water** and **2 tablespoons of Epsom salts**; apply directly to the wounded skin using a soaked, clean cloth.

♥

19) Bruising Solution

It may be hard to believe that Epsom salt can even help with bruises - but it can. Create a soothing bath soak for the bruised areas with a combination of **2 cups of Epsom salt** and **1 tub-full of warm water**. This will help speed up the recovery process by promoting blood flow, which will sooner decrease the appearance of your injuries.

Alternatively, you can also soak a cloth in a mixture of **2 tablespoons of Epsom salts** and **1 cup of cold water**, and apply it directly over the bruise.

♥

20) Hangover Soak

Hangover? Hey, we've all been there! Before you go and grab that greasy take-away meal, try this hangover cure instead, courtesy of trusty Epsom salts.

Hangovers are a result of alcohol toxicity in the body.

Help get rid of those toxins by soaking in **a tub-full of warm water** and **2 cups of Epsom salts** for 15-30 minutes. For an even bigger boost, pour some other revitalizing ingredients into your Epsom salt bath, such as **essential oils like tea tree, lavender, or lemon**. The magnesium in the salts will help you detoxify while the essential oils will stimulate your senses and clear a foggy mind.

21) Jet-Lag Soak

Jet-lag is horrible; that wear and tear on the body and mind is a killer, isn't it? Rather than endure the tiredness and fogginess, use the power of minerals in Epsom salts to speed up your recovery. This will help rejuvenate your muscles and joints and help the body restore its natural energy levels. The magnesium sulfate wakes up the natural healing capacity in your body and also gets rid of any stiffness, aches and pains that may result from sitting in a cramped plane or car. On top of that, Epsom salts can help normalize your sleeping patterns when bathing before bedtime.

For 15 minutes, soak yourself in **a tub-full of warm water** and **2 cups of Epsom salts**. You will surely be in for a good night's rest!

22) Poison Ivy Compress

Poison ivy releases a sticky substance called *urushiol*

(an allergen). When this allergen comes in contact with the skin, a person may experience minimal to severe reactions such as rashes and blisters. Are you prepared for when this happens?

Never fear, Epsom salts have you covered! For quick and easy poison ivy relief, just make a compress to apply to your irritated skin. Simply soak a clean cloth in **a cup of cold water** mixed with **2 tablespoons of Epsom salts**. Pat over affected area and leave for a few minutes.

Dr. Joe Matusic, a pediatrician from Charleston West Virginia, states: *'Anything that itches and burns the skin, Epsom salt can cure'*.

Epsom salts can positively impact many facets of our day-to-day lives. Boosting health from the inside out; be sure to take advantage of these super simple yet highly effective remedies.

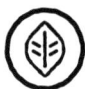

CHAPTER 3

Epsom Salt for Health

Perhaps it is its association with our grandmothers that made us hesitant about using these age-old Epsom salt remedies. The reality is that most of us are just not aware of how great Epsom salts can be for our overall health. There are many healthful benefits to incorporating Epsom salts into our daily or weekly routine, and best of all, it is so easy. It is a reliable, affordable and safe way to relieve common ailments and boost your body's overall wellbeing.

Health Remedies

The following remedies use Epsom salts for a variety of health concerns and conditions. You have already discovered a variety of sea bath recipes and cosmetic and first aid uses, but now it is time to explore even more possibilities for your inner health. Even medical professionals boast the benefits of this miraculous mineral.

If you suffer from any pain, arthritis or cramped muscles, then you will definitely benefit from Epsom salts. When the mineral is absorbed through the skin, it works instantaneously to relieve soreness and helps you feel better from the inside out. This is because the magnesium ions in the product separate themselves from the Epsom salt molecules – the ions then work to ease your cramps from stress, work, or physical activity by encouraging more serotonin production in the body. The magnesium in the ions also work to produce more white blood cells, which help your body feel renewed, refreshed, and revitalized.

When cold and flu season strikes, do you rush to your drugstore for a whole stock of medications and remedies? Well, if you want something that is more natural and just as effective, then put down the packages of cough syrups and decongestants and pick up some Epsom salts instead. These little guys are loaded with beneficial properties that are welcomed when cold and flus attack.

As previously mentioned, Epsom salts are wonderful for relieving aches and pains, which definitely come hand-in-hand with cold-weather viruses and the flu. When you are relieved of body aches, you can fall asleep easier and get the rest your body so desperately needs.

Epsom salts can be used at the first sign of sickness; soaking yourself in a detoxifying bath is not only relaxing, but can serve as a proactive step in warding off prolonged illness. The sooner, the better. Epsom salt baths help your body speed up the process of 'vasodilation', which is when your white blood cells produce more rapidly to help fight-off nasty viruses. While your white blood cells get to work, your immune system will become strengthened as a result of magnesium sulfate's alkaline elements.

Back when N1H1 (Swine Flu) was a serious concern, doctors and medical professionals suggested that patients soak in an Epsom salt bath so that they could better relieve the body aches and pains associated with the virus. Magnesium is known to get the lactic acid (which causes pain) moving and flowing out of the muscles, so even healthy individuals can benefit from a soak, particularly after a workout.

Who knew that this unsuspecting mineral could pack such a punch?

♥

23) Soothing Salt Bath for Aches & Pains

Cramping up? After a tough workout, or if you simply experience troublesome aches and pains, this soothing bath will relieve your muscle pain and joint inflammation. Fill your tub with **warm water** (to promote circulation) and mix in **1/2 cup of Epsom salts**.

Need to relax? Then add **a few drops of lavender oil**, or alternatively, you can use **chamomile essential oil** for added anti-inflammatory effects.

NOTE: You can also resort to bathing with Epsom salts using the recipes we have covered in chapter 2.

♥

24) Flu-Fighting Soak

Reap the immune-strengthening benefits of Epsom salt by simply soaking yourself in this flu-fighting remedy. It is simple, relaxing, and effective.

Ingredients:

• Epsom salts, 1 cup

• Baking soda, 1/2 cup

• Sliced or powdered ginger, 1 Tablespoon *(a natural decongestant)*

• Warm water, one bathtub-full

• Essential oil of your choice, 5-10 drops *(eucalyptus also works as an effective decongestant)*

Directions:

1) Add all the ingredients to the tub.

2) Soak body in bath for at least 20 minutes.

♥

25) Indigestion Relief

No one likes to admit that they suffer from indigestion, but it is actually quite a common malady. The food you ingest interacts with your stomach acid, which breaks down the food for easier digestion. Sometimes acidic food can slip back up into the esophagus causing varying levels of discomfort.

Fortunately, there is a natural and affordable solution. Yes, you guessed it: Epsom salts. They serve as a natural antacid, neutralizing your stomach acid so you feel less burn and discomfort. Simply mix **a cup of warm water** with **1 tablespoon of Epsom salt** – you may also add the Epsom salt to **a cup of peppermint tea** to help soothe even further. Dissolve and drink slowly.

26) Beverage to Regulate Blood Sugar

Did you know that Epsom salts are great for regulating blood sugar and helping with insulin resistance? Studies have shown that low magnesium can play a role in insulin resistance and diabetes. With an occasional dose of the minerals in Epsom salts, you can help regulate your blood sugar levels and improve insulin resistance, in conjunction with a healthy, whole food, plant-based diet.

This beverage is made by simply mixing **a cup of warm water** and **1 tablespoon of Epsom salt**; dissolve and drink slowly, followed by another glass of water. Consume this beverage only on occasion and consult your doctor to ensure Epsom salt is suitable for you.

Alternatively you can enjoy a simple Epsom salt foot soak **(2 tablespoons of Epsom salt with warm water)** to absorb magnesium through the skin – but first ensure your feet have no cuts, sores or irritation.

♥

27) Sleepy-Time Bath

Having trouble getting some shut-eye? Tired of counting sheep or watching mindless infomercials on late-night television? Good thing Epsom salts can help.

For better sleep, just soak in a warm and wonderful Epsom salt bath. This is a great way to get both kids and adults ready for bedtime. So, how does it work?

When our bodies endure the stressful daily grind day after day, magnesium seeps out of our system, causing a deficiency. As mentioned, magnesium works to produce more serotonin, which tells the adrenaline in our bodies to 'chill out'.

So, soak yourself in a magnesium-rich Epsom salt bath before bedtime to replenish your body's magnesium levels and bring your body into a relaxed and calmed state – **1/2 cup of Epsom salt** to **a tub-full of warm water**. Add a few drops of your favorite relaxing **essential oils (such as lavender or chamomile)** for added tranquility.

♥

28) Arthritis-Easing Soak

Arthritis can be debilitating – the chronic pain and inflammation can really take a toll on our mind and body. Using Epsom salts to ease stiffness in your joints is a great way to reduce arthritis symptoms. Epsom salts allow your body to take in more oxygen, which helps to ease inflammation, as well as prevent your arteries from hardening.

You can soak your entire body in this mixture **(2 cups of Epsom salt in 1 tub-full of warm water)**, or you may also use a large bowl to soak an arthritis-ridden area of your body, such as hands or feet **(2 tablespoons of Epsom salt in warm water)**. This remedy is much cheaper and more satisfying than commercial products and solutions.

♥

29) Constipation Reliever

Did you know that Epsom salts work as a saline laxative? Relieve your constipation woes by dissolving **1 teaspoon of Epsom salt** in **1 cup of warm water** and drink it straight down, followed by a glass of water – you may add a dash of lemon juice to taste. This mixture can be consumed twice per day, 4 hours apart, for 4 days.

The reason this works is because Epsom salt belongs to the laxative group, *oral hyperosmotic*, due to its magnesium and sulfate components. Upon ingestion, the minerals help to move water through the colon and loosen waste matter, making it easier to pass a bowel movement. The magnesium can also trigger muscle contractions that can push waste out of the colon.

♥

30) Bath for Muscles & Nerves

When you suffer from muscle and nerve cramping or pain, it can be hard to go about your daily activities. The magnesium sulfate in Epsom salts regulate and improve the capabilities of enzymes in the body, particularly those that address fluid retention (which can lead to decreased nerve and muscle function). Epsom salts can also help your body utilize calcium and sends signals to your brain to activate different chemical functions.

All you need to do is soak in some Epsom salts a few days per week. Simply mix **2 cups of Epsom salts** in **a bathtub-full of warm water**, and soak for 15-45 minutes. After just a few soaks, expect to notice an improvement in your muscle and nerve function.

❤️

31) Blood Circulation Boosting Bath

So you now know that an Epsom salt bath is great for reducing the inflammation associated with arthritis, the aches and pains of a cold or flu and any muscle and nerve discomfort. Let's add yet another benefit, shall we?

Get into an Epsom salt bathtub for a boost to your blood circulation. With its high levels of magnesium and sulfate, Epsom salts can boost the circulation of blood in your body while lowering your blood pressure. Just soak (using any of the bath recipes in this book) for 20-40 minutes, and you are in for a handful of hearty benefits such as: improved arterial elasticity, prevention of blood clots, reduction of plaque buildups and lessened damage to arterial walls. In simple terms, you can improve your overall cardiovascular health with regular Epsom salt baths. Include a few drops of geranium or rosemary essential oils for added circulatory effects.

❤️

32) Gout Soother

If you are dealing with gout, then you know how much of a pain it can be. Much like arthritis, gout leaves your joints feeling inflamed and achy because there is too much uric acid in the body. With its detoxifying properties, Epsom salt can be an absolute savior.

Through flushing out the excess uric acid (that usually is purged through urine), Epsom salts work with joint proteins to clear out the build-up. The magnesium in the salts will work to ease the inflammatory symptoms while helping your nerves regularly distribute electrolytes.

In a large bowl or foot-tub, **fill with warm water** and mix in **2 tablespoons of Epsom salt**. You may also add **a few drops of peppermint essential oil** to help cool and ease the pain. Soak your hands or feet for 15-30 minutes and experience the soothing relief. Try it as often as you need for a quick solution to any swelling and discomfort.

♥

33) Magnesium Mineral Booster

This next tip is a no-brainer. We talked about how many Americans are deficient in magnesium, an essential element that our bodies need. We also know that taking a bath in Epsom salts can help boost your magnesium levels in a safe and healthy way. But have you ever wondered why magnesium is so important? Some background information about this element may give you more insight into why it is crucial to keep your body's magnesium levels in check.

While magnesium may not be a mineral that we tend to keep an eye on, it plays a pivotal role in the way our body functions. In fact, magnesium is present in more than 300 different chemical interactions that take place in our bodies. A lack of magnesium could lead to decreased energy levels, tension and anxiety, restless joints and limbs, weaker bones, a higher risk of heart disease and lower stamina. Even your heart's blood vessels and arteries need magnesium in order to function properly. Don't be complacent – have a blood test to determine whether you are magnesium deficient, or you'll never know until it's too late.

Since magnesium can be depleted from the soil our fresh produce is grown in today, it can be hard for most individuals around the world to get enough of it. We are lucky enough to have access to this essential mineral through a variety of means, including **beans, whole grains, almonds, sesame seeds, sunflower seeds, dark chocolate (dairy free)**, and of course, **Epsom salt**. If your doctor tells you that your magnesium levels are low, try incorporating those magnesium-rich foods into your diet, and also take the time to give your body (and your mind) some rest with the relaxing magnesium-rich bath remedies within this book. Bathing twice or thrice per week is the perfect way to start replenishing your body.

Weight Loss

Who doesn't love to hear the words 'weight loss'? However, this goal can be a slippery slope, especially with the onslaught of marketing claims and products that we see and hear about everywhere! Now though, when combined with a diet rich in healthy plant foods, you can be assured that this natural mineral that has been trusted for hundreds of years will aid you in achieving your weight loss goals. Take a look at these weight-loss benefits; you may decide to try out these remedies to help achieve your desired results.

Cellulite. It is simply a fact of life for men and women of various ages and backgrounds. While it can be hard to escape cellulite completely, you can really get a leg up on it (no pun intended) with the help of Epsom salts. I know what you're thinking: 'Impossible!' But, hear me out.

Epsom salts are great for firming and evening out skin tone, and are effective in cleansing and extracting toxins stored in your body's fat cells – so it makes sense that this mineral can help lessen and smooth the appearance of cellulite. Soaking in an Epsom salt bath or using a homemade cellulite-busting scrub may beat those expensive, upmarket lotions and potions.

While you kick cellulite in the butt, why not get in on the weight-loss advantages of an Epsom salt soak? Magnesium detoxifies the body while regulating the functions of your muscles, nerves and hundreds of enzymes. Additionally, sulfate works to keep your skin looking fresh and hydrated and it also boosts collagen production so that you look more radiant without the use of heavy creams and lotions.

What does all of this mean for weight loss? *A build up of toxins in the body play a role in fat cell buildup.* When bathing in a warm soak of Epsom salt, your pores will open up to help these toxins get flushed out, assisting in the role of weight loss. This, along with a whole food, plant-based diet will help detox your body on a holistic level – from the inside out. With the cosmetic benefits of Epsom salts and a nutrient-filled diet of plant-based foods, your outer appearance will remain revitalized and refreshed and your inner health will be optimal.

♥

34) Cellulite-Busting Scrub

Who would have guessed that adding Epsom salts to your daily body scrub could reap cellulite-busting benefits as well as smooth, firm skin?

Ingredients:
- Epsom salts, 2 Tablespoons
- Maple syrup, 4 Tablespoons
- Brown sugar, 1 Tablespoon

Optional:
- Lemon juice, 1 Tablespoon

Directions:

1) Mix maple syrup and brown sugar. You can add some zest by simply mixing in a tablespoon of lemon juice.

2) Once combined, mix in the Epsom salts.

3) Massage onto any problem areas. Leave for a few minutes before rinsing with warm water.

♥

35) Detoxifying Weight Loss Soak

Along with Epsom salt, baking soda, ginger and grapefruit essential oil will amp up the detoxing process, helping open up the pores to make you sweat and promote weight-loss.

Ingredients:

• Epsom salts, 1 Tablespoon

• Baking soda, 1 Tablespoon

• Sliced or powdered ginger, 1 Tablespoon **OR** Apple Cider Vinegar, 1 cup

• Warm water, one tubful

• Grapefruit essential oil, 5-10 drops

Directions:

1) Add Epsom salts to bathtub, allow to dissolve. Add the baking soda, ginger (or ACV) and essential oil and mix well.

2) Soak entire body in bath for at least 15 minutes.

3) Since this will be a regular regimen, gradually increase the measurement of Epsom salt until you reach 2 cups.

With this being said, these remedies should not replace a sensible diet and regular exercise regimen – Epsom salt will give you a little extra help to boost your progress. All of these Epsom salt applications are natural, effective and a breeze to implement into your daily life.

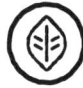

CHAPTER 4

Epsom Salt for Home & Garden

We have already delved into how to use Epsom salts to take care of your mind and body, both inside and out, but what about caring for your surroundings – like your home and garden? If you weren't thrilled enough already with the many uses for Epsom salts, there are still more! You'll definitely get your money's worth and then some.

In this chapter, we will explore how you can use Epsom salts to improve the look and feel of your home as well as your outdoor areas and gardens.

Gardening

First off, we will address how to use Epsom salts to benefit and nourish your garden. Whether you have a huge plot of land or just a flower box on your windowsill, you can give your greenery a refresher with this versatile ingredient.

Just as Epsom salts are healthy for our bodies, they are also healthful for plants and conditioning garden soil. The sulfate component in this sustainable mineral encourages plants to grow and blossom, and plays a key role in the germination and growth of seeds. It also aids in the process of chlorophyll production and strengthens the cell walls of fruits and nuts, while aiding in the plants' intake of nitrogen, phosphorus, and sulfur.

Just like our bodies can be deficient in minerals, soils can be too. Both the magnesium and sulfate found in Epsom salt are necessary nutritional elements for the health of many plants. Plant varieties that are particularly susceptible to nutritional deficiencies from magnesium and sulfate include; *tomatoes, peppers, and rose flowers*. If you notice your plants or crops have yellowing or curling leaves, slow growth, a bitter taste or little to no sweetness (in the case of fruit), then they may very well be lacking in these important minerals. Increasing the production of vitamins, amino acids, plant protein and enzymes within crops (such as broccoli, for example) results in tastier, robust flavors.

If you discover your soil has a low pH level (or a pH higher than 7), this may be an indication that your soil is lacking in essential magnesium. This can result when other minerals, such as calcium and potassium, take center stage and leave very little room for magnesium to be absorbed into the plants' roots. You can determine the pH levels in your soil with a soil testing kit from your local garden center or hardware store.

Epsom salts are highly soluble and don't build up in soil over time, making them the perfect nutritional solution. You can simply dissolve Epsom salt in water, or even mix them in with your regular soil spray – you will be sure to see improvements in no time!

36) Fertilizer Spray

Why use processed, chemical laden fertilizers? Fertilizing your plants just got a whole lot easier with the help of all-natural Epsom salts. Many seasoned gardeners claim that adding Epsom salt to their flowers and foliage improves the vibrancy and strength of their blooms. Try out this foliar spray for happier, healthier plants.

Dilute **2 tablespoons of Epsom salt per 1 gallon (4L) of water** *(or around 1 teaspoon of Epsom salt per 1 water-filled spray bottle)*. Allow the mixture to dissolve and transfer into a spray bottle or a tank sprayer. Spritz directly onto your plants once per month in replacement of a regular watering.

NOTE: Do not over-do spraying and be mindful that Epsom salts can cause leaf burn if applied to plants on a hot, sunny day.

37) Pest and Insect Deterrent

So now you know how to fertilize your plants, but what about those cheeky pests that chomp away at them? Try this Epsom salt remedy for a non-toxic insect and pest deterrent that won't leave your garden laden with chemicals.

Take **a handful of Epsom salt** and place them directly on or nearby areas where slugs and pests crawl or stray – *and that's it*. This solution will naturally deter raccoons, slugs, mosquitos and other creepy crawlies without the use of harmful chemical pesticides.

♥

38) Healthy Roses, Tomatoes & Peppers

We mentioned earlier that tomatoes, peppers and roses are especially prone to magnesium deficiencies. Well there is a way to help those plants and crops make it through the entire planting and harvesting season – this solution may even help to eliminate that end-of-season rot and decay.

The directions are super simple – you can even ask the kids to help out. Just use **1 tablespoon of Epsom salt** per **1 gallon (4L) of water**. Mix well and pour the solution directly into the surrounding soil every few weeks. In a hurry? Then just scoop a small handful and sprinkle it at the base of your plants.

♥

39) Fruit Tree Fertilizer

When it comes to planting and taking care of fruit trees, these plants require lots of time and patience – and when the season ends for some crops, these fruit trees need to keep on going. So ensure that your fruit trees stay strong and lush by feeding them the nutrients contained in Epsom salts. You may even find the fruit tastes sweeter and looks healthier too.

What's great about this solution is the convenience – a

little goes a long way. Can you believe all you need to do to make a lasting impact on your fruit trees is give them some Epsom salt *a few times a year*? Per 9 square feet of soil, simply mix in **2 tablespoons** of Epsom salts (especially near the root area), and voila!

♥

40) Luscious Lawns

Wouldn't it be nice to have grass that always looks green, thick, and oh so lush? Just take advantage of this simple trick. This Epsom salt application aids in germination and seed health – roots will grow stronger and won't easily succumb to heavy treading or intense weather.

Use **3 pounds of Epsom salt per 1,250 square feet of grass** and evenly disperse using a lawn spreader – hose down afterward. Alternatively if you wish to cover a smaller area, mix **2 tablespoons of Epsom salt per 1 gallon (4L) of water** and spritz directly over the grass using a tank sprayer. Use this treatment regularly for a luscious lawn your neighbors will envy!

♥

41) Easy Stump Removal Aid

If you have ever tried to clear away tree stumps from your property, you know that it can leave your garden looking like a disaster zone! Well, Epsom salts can help make this process much easier by getting to the 'root' of the problem without spending thousands of dollars having it professionally removed.

Drill several holes into the top of the stump (about 3-4 inches apart). Pour **dry Epsom salt** directly into the holes to fill them, followed by **a slow pouring of water** until salt is moistened. Epsom salts are great moisture absorbers, as we already know, and will help dry out the stump so it is easier to remove. If not successful the first time, simply repeat the process every 3 weeks.

♥

42) Compost Deodorizer

Composting is a wonderful, environmentally friendly way to add nutrient-rich plant materials back into nature, but unfortunately we are left to endure the issue of compost odor, which can attract flies and pests to your garden and home. Try using this simple trick to mask odors and absorb bacteria whilst adding extra nutrients to your compost.

To begin with, simply sprinkle 3 cups of Epsom salts over your compost heap and distribute evenly. As you add more compost to your pile, you may add in a few more tablespoons each week to maintain a stench-free garden. Visitors may not even notice your compost supply at first sniff!

Household

Finally, it's time to discover the wonderful uses of Epsom salts in your very own home! I understand how tiresome it can be to keep your house looking pristine and spotless. Fortunately, Epsom salts can make cleaning easier, healthier and more convenient for you and your family. Whether you're scrubbing your bathroom and kitchen, keeping utensils and dishes sparkling, or preserving the vibrancy of your carpet – there are loads of uses for Epsom salts in your home. And best of all, it is a non-toxic, inexpensive alternative to harmful, commercial products.

43) Tile and Grout Cleaner

We just don't have time to scrub all day long, but this easy-breezy combination will help speed up the process; an absolute essential for your bathroom, kitchen and more.

Ingredients:

• Epsom salts, 1 cup

• Liquid Castille soap, 1 cup

• Baking soda, 1/2 cup

Directions:

1) Combine Epsom salts, baking soda, and soap; stir together thoroughly.

2) Apply to tile or grout and let sit for 15 minutes.

3) Scrub using clockwise motion.

4) Rinse thoroughly.

44) Spic-&-Span Pot & Pan Cleaner

Have you ever slaved over the kitchen sink in the desperate hopes of getting that burnt pasta sauce or cooked-on pancake off of the pan? Even ever-convenient dishwashers just don't cut it at times. The next time you have food stuck to your pots and pans, grab a trusty bag of Epsom salts. The crystals will do the hard work for you by creating an abrasive texture to scrape off residue without leaving your cookware tarnished or discolored.

Just add approximately **1/4 tablespoon of Epsom salts** directly into your pots and pans, let sit a few minutes before adding warm water, and scrub well.

45) House-Plant Refresher

We discovered how to care for plants, trees and flowers in your outdoor garden; but how about indoor house-plants? They too can benefit from a dose of Epsom salts. Not only will your blooms stay fresh; they will look healthier and grow faster.

In **a water-filled spray bottle**, mix in **1 teaspoon of Epsom salt.** Spray onto your plants once per month in replacement of a regular watering. Spritzing this solution directly onto plants is a great way for the nutrients in Epsom salt to be readily and easily absorbed.

♥

46) Rust Remover

Rust stains can occur just about anywhere in the home, such as your kitchen, bathroom or garage. Luckily, combining Epsom salt with a simple ingredient from your kitchen will help those rust stains vanish before your eyes.

Ingredients:
• Epsom salts, 4 Tablespoons
• Juice of half a lemon
• Water, 1 Tablespoon

Directions:
1) Mix Epsom salts and lemon juice together.

2) Add just enough water so that the mixture has a paste consistency.

3) Rub on rust and allow to dry.

4) Gently buff area with a dry, clean cloth or rag.

♥

47) Carpet & Rug Cleaner

If you've considered replacing your rugs or carpets because they look as though they have lost their luster, try these Epsom salt tricks before you commit to that big purchase. You can remove stains and brighten up your carpet with a simple solution of Epsom salt and water – you can even use this mixture on fabric curtains.

Mix **1 cup of Epsom salt** to **1/2 gallon (2L) of water** then take a clean cloth and soak it in the solution. Wring out the cloth and use it to spot-clean any stains – you may also use an old toothbrush to gently scrub stubborn areas. For stained curtains and rags, simply wash them with an Epsom salt solution using the same measurements (you may multiply measurements if necessary) and rinse well.

48) Hole-in-the-Wall Filler

Oops! Don't just cover it with a poster. It has never been easier to repair a hole or chip in your drywall or plaster walls – this paste can be whipped up in a jiffy.

Ingredients:

• Epsom salts, 2 Tablespoons

• Cornstarch, 2 Tablespoons

• Water, 5 Tablespoons *(enough to make a paste)*

Directions:

1) Combine Epsom salt and cornstarch and mix well.

2) Add enough water so that a thick paste is formed.

3) Apply the salt paste to the fill the holes; smooth with a spatula.

49) Fabric Softener

Rather than splurge on expensive fabric softeners, try this two-ingredient fabric softener that is all-natural and super easy to make at home, saving you loads of money in the long run.

To keep your clothes soft and fresh, simply use **1/4 cup of Epsom salt** per load of laundry, and **a dash of your favorite essential oil** for a pleasing scent. Really, it doesn't get easier and cheaper than this. Not only will fabrics feel softer, it will also brighten colors and remove stubborn stains!

50) Washing Machine Cleanser

Soap scum, grime, dirt and bacteria can build up in our washing machines over time. There is nothing more frustrating than washing clothes only to have them covered in residue and looking even dirtier than before! Try this quick trick to cleanse and remove build-up from your washing machine.

Fill your empty washing machine with hot water and add **1 cup of Epsom salt**, plus **1 quart (1L) of white vinegar**. Allow the machine to cycle for just a few minutes, then pause and let steep for a few of hours to allow the solution to remove odors and break down residue. Next, complete a full wash and rinse cycle.

If you have a front-load washer, add the same mixture into the drum and simply run through a hot cycle.

Using a cloth soaked in Epsom salt and water, open the washer lid and wipe down the inside blades, filter or dispenser drawer to remove any lingering gunk. You may run your washing machine through one more cycle to ensure all grime is gone. Use this method every few months or when required.

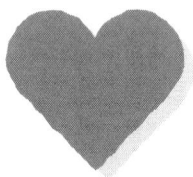

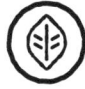

THANK YOU

At long last, you have discovered the many ways to incorporate Epsom salts into your daily life and routine. Thank you for purchasing this book and exploring the many methods that will enable you to utilize this natural and effective ingredient for a variety of every day tasks. Who knew that this naturally occurring mineral would be helpful in so many ways?

While there are many uses, you may have come across a few of your own favorites that you are looking forward to trying out. Whether you utilize all or just a few of these Epsom salt tips and tricks, I hope that you find them to be a versatile and helpful aid for your home and health.

I love keeping in touch with my readers, so be sure to stay connected with the *Carma Books* community and email list for special offers and more books on holistic and natural living.

Until next time, I wish you a beautiful journey in happiness and health.

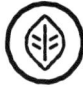

A WORD FROM THE PUBLISHER

Hi, I'm Carmen, a holistic health geek with a passion for health, herbalism, natural remedies, as well as whole-food and plant-based lifestyles. After resolving various health issues I have struggled with for many years, I aim to inspire and help improve your health and longevity by sharing the tireless hours of research and valuable information I have discovered throughout my journey. Through the power of nutrition and lifestyle, with an evidence-based approach, I believe you can achieve your health and wellness goals.

If you enjoyed this book, I would love to hear how it has benefited you and invite you to leave a short review on Amazon - your valuable feed-back is always appreciated!

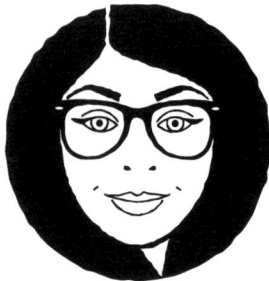

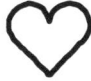

You are invited to to join our **Free Book Club**
mailing list. Sign up via our website to receive
special offers *and* ***free for a limited time***
Health & Wellness eBooks!

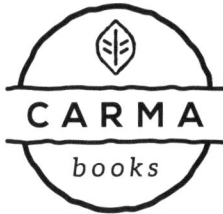

CARMA

books

'A conscious approach to health & wellness'

carmabooks.com

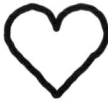

THANK YOU